# LYME DISEASE

# NON-MEDICAL DIAGNOSIS AND TREATMENT

How I Kicked Chronic Lyme disease in One Year for Pennies

# Terms and Conditions

# Table of Contents

# Introduction

I ran an engineering firm, designed modifications on off-road motorcycles, and raced them in International competition winning many 1st places, medals, etc... My wife of 23 years got Cancer at the age of 38.

We knew nothing about health except to eat what they told us was a balanced diet and exercise properly. We didn't know that the balanced diet everyone was eating was not proper nutrition.

The doctor recommended chemotherapy and radiation. Naturally, frightened as we were, we let them do it and the doctor managed to kill her in less than a year.

I knew there was something wrong with that picture, so I started putting as much effort into health studies as I had into motorsports.

I enrolled at the College of Life Science in Austin, Texas. A few years later I received my doctorate in natural nutrition, and I've never stopped researching the causes of our health problems.

I contracted Lyme disease about 14 years ago. Six years later, it showed up as several physical problems during a stressful situation. Since I had no tick bite, it was three more painful years before Lyme was even considered.

The purpose of this small book is to alert you to the hidden epidemic - Lyme disease. I am letting you know, whatever name they may put on your diagnosis, you can probably kick it out of your body for about $25.00 using a certain alternative product.

Almost no health problem is a death sentence. We are brainwashed to think sickness - not wellness. Just because you contract, a dis-ease doesn't mean you have to die from it. If you research other alternative remedies, what others have used to overcome illness you might have a better chance. And if you are not pushed into traditional (deadly) treatment with pharmaceuticals you might have a better chance of getting well by improving your immune system.

Lasting health is built from building up the inside health and not by poisoning your body back to health. The conventional health system is about administering drugs and controlling disease. Alternative health is about correcting the nutritional deficiencies, eating more organic foods and juicing fresh and raw foods.

We also found it useful to use a broad spectrum pathogen killer to rid the body of bacteria, viruses and fungus.

For an interesting point of view concerning cancer, from the book: "The Only Answer to Cancer" one of the leading authors on cancer said, "Most people will have cancer 5 to 6 times in a lifetime, and they will never know it because the body takes care of it automatically."

It's only after the immune system gets overwhelmed that cancer or most anything else can become a killer disease.

# *Lyme Disease Non Medical Diagnosis and Treatment*

How I Kicked Chronic Lyme disease in One Year for Pennies

# Chapter 1:

## *How'd I Get Lyme Disease?*

---

# Synopsis

This chapter is covering the unusual way I got Lyme disease, what causes it and why it's seldom diagnosed correctly.

You will also learn what stress has to do with getting sick with a serious disease and the symptoms Lyme causes, and how Lyme Disease can hide for years in your body.

A little-known fact:
**Lyme Disease is highly contagious.**

# How'd I Get Lyme Disease?

I had active Lyme Disease for nine years before I figured out what was wrong. Neither any doctor nor I thought of Lyme Disease because I didn't get a tick bite, and everybody believed the propaganda of the deer tick being the only way you get the disease.

People who live in the city usually do not go into deer woods and cannot believe they might have Lyme Disease. Their doctors have the same mindset and do not consider such a disease and do not diagnosis it either.

**A very smart bacteria is the cause of Lyme Disease**

Not only is it hard to detect but also it is a smart bacteria that can avoid the traditional treatment with antibiotics. "Lyme bacteria have evolved ways to escape the effects of antibiotics and evade the immune system." Reports Leo Galland, M.D

# A mosquito bit me, not the deer tick

I wondered about the mosquito bite I had gotten about ten years before. It didn't go away for months. Since then, I've found out you can get Lyme from any biting insect and from close contact with any person or pet that has it.

## What Are the Other Names OF Lyme Disease?

Lyme Disease is caused by a tiny corkscrew-shaped bacterium called Spirochete (Pronounced *Spiro-kete*). Spirochetes are spiral shaped (snake-like) bacteria, gram-negative, capable of spontaneously and independently traveling, sized from 3 to 500 micrometers long.

## This same type of bacteria causes 3 well-known communicable diseases:

- **Syphilis**
- **Relapsing fever**
- **Lyme Disease (Borreliosis).**

Both Syphilis and Lyme can cause a range of symptoms that belong to over 300 different diseases. So, Lyme Disease is seldom diagnosed correctly because the patient may not have been bitten by any insect, let alone a tick. Therefore, the idea of Lyme disease as a possibility hardly ever enters the mind of an MD. Since it is a hidden epidemic meaning, there is no media news; the average people do not know they might easily get it from various means of which I will soon explain.

It might be interesting to note that everyone in a family and even the pets can be sick with the disease, and each one can show entirely different symptoms.

The main reason for the many symptoms is that these bacteria set up their colonies in the weakest points in each body they invade. Therefore, each person or animal with these bacteria may seem to have a completely different disease.

**The many faces of the same disease**

My body appeared to have Fibromyalgia and rheumatoid arthritis while my wife, Taylore, who got it from me, had severe digestive problems. Because of the exceptionally different symptoms, very few doctors, either natural or allopathic, would ever guess we both had the same disease. The upshot is that many families all have Lyme disease, and they are taking different medications. The sad thing is none of them are probably taking a remedy that addresses the real problem. There is only one proven solution that completely takes care of the problem, and we will tell all about it soon.

**Three forms of Borrelia burgdorferi, the spirochete that causes Lyme Disease**

The Spirochete can hide in your body for years without being noticed and suddenly causes trouble after some stressful event.
It changes back and forth between 3 different forms therefore making it difficult to diagnosis because it looks like three dissimilar organisms.

**The three forms of spirochetes are:**

- **Spiral shape** - like a corkscrew or tiny snake
- **Cell wall deficient** - means it does not have a cell wall in this stage. It is jelly-like.
- **Encysted** or encapsulated in a shell - it can form a cover around itself impervious to antibiotics.

Remember this same little bacteria changes shapes and forms to hide from medications. It acts like it has consciousness; it is a smart bug, and it forms colonies in areas it likes.

**Spirochetes are said to behave more intelligently than other bacteria**

Some researchers think they are in many ways more evolved than other bacteria. They are said to almost show signs of animal-like behavior. Borrelia bacteria have a good transportation system, both forward and backward, where they can travel quickly all over the body. Borrelia is a genus of bacteria of the spirochete family. Other bacteria are non-motile, but the Borrelia have a distinct advantage in that they can move anywhere they, please picking the best locations for their colonies.

**Results of the Spirochete Colonies I felt were:**
- Overall weakness in my body
- Deep muscle pain
- Aching muscles and joints
- Loss of all muscle strength
- Weakness in the arms and legs

- Sleep Apnea

I had an inability to get up off the floor without help. It was mysterious because I had been so strong all my life.

I couldn't find out what was making my muscles so weak and painful-to-the-bone, including intense joint pain of osteoarthritis in my hands that also included my whole body? I couldn't even lift my legs or get up off the floor if I got down. I was so weak. After checking symptoms for several diseases, I finally found an alternative doctor who examined the symptoms and decided that I must have Lyme disease and did the test.

He recommended some natural products because we researched in several places on the Internet that antibiotics don't work well with the Lyme bacteria. They hide in an encasement until you stop taking the antibiotic and then come back and start multiplying again. We needed something that would instantly work so the little critters did not have time to hide, or encase themselves. All this research has lead us to our discovery that we will soon share with you.

The general experience of Lyme Disease sufferers goes something like this man's testimonial.

*"I became symptomatic with Lyme disease in February of 1999. At this time, I had thought for all practical purposes my life was over. Many days I felt that I could not even get out of bed. For those who don't know Lyme disease is an extremely debilitating as well as it is a difficult disease to diagnose and to treat. The Lyme spirochete is a hardier organism than the typical bacterium the conventional medicine arena is used to seeing and treating. The adaptability of the spirochete leads to infinite amount of problems with conventional treatment. The list of symptoms I experienced is endless including, joint pain, migraine headaches, memory loss, muscle twitches, extreme fatigue, abdominal discomfort, brain fog, etc... Basically anyone with full blown late stage Lyme disease is not living; they are merely suffering in a conscious coma. "*
By Jim P. who eventually recovered from Lyme disease.

# Chapter 2:

*A Well Hidden Epidemic?*

---

# Synopsis

In this chapter, you will find out if you live in an area where you could contract Lyme disease.

You will also understand why it is seldom diagnosed correctly and the magnitude of the epidemic.

Discover how the words you think and say about a disease can heal you or make your disease worse and make it a lifetime battle.

Learn the origin of the name of this close relative to syphilis, which belies its seriousness.

# A Well Hidden Epidemic?

It is an epidemic that is not even acknowledged to exist. The CDC seems to be under-reporting its seriousness. Doctors are still telling patients who live in cities that a person cannot possibly have Lyme if they live in a city.

It's still called a tick-borne disease even though you can get it from any biting insect or any body fluid from anyone who has it including your pets. Don't forget licking, sneezing, sweating, kissing, by blood transfusions and, of course; sex transfers bodily fluids that may contain the bacteria of Lyme Disease.

We are wondering why the media is still reporting that it is only carried by a certain deer tick and that tick is only in certain states? One doctor told a lady that she could not have Lyme Disease because she lived in Georgia. She had 10 of the known symptoms.

Once we found out that we had Lyme Disease, we started to search out various treatments. Some authorities will say that it is incurable. From reading testimonials on the various Lyme Disease forums, we noticed comments that hundreds of men and women have been suffering from terrible symptoms for years spending up to one hundred thousand dollars.

We prayed to God for a solution and were lucky to find Chlorine Dioxide to get rid of the Lyme disease bacteria we'd had almost ten years. You notice I didn't say we cured it. The Lyme disease was very healthy and didn't need "curing". The body needed a curing.

**The Words You Use**
Most of us say, "We want to cure a disease" when we really want it to be gone. Since our words are LAW in our bodies, saying we want to "cure our disease" simply makes the disease stronger and us weaker!

Remember to love and support your body. Appreciate and be thankful for your wonderful body! Some people don't pay any attention to their body or what they feed it until it gets sick. Then they curse it for being weak or sick. Treat your body like a fine machine and a good friend!

**What Is Lyme Disease?**

If you were to use computer terminology to describe Lyme disease, you would probably call it Syphilis 3.0. So how did this close relative of Syphilis get an innocent sounding name, like Lyme disease?

The first time it was diagnosed as a distinct disease separate from Syphilis was in Lyme, Connecticut. Lyme is very close to Plum Island, where the government does biological warfare experiments and creates new germs.

**Regardless of how it came about, Lyme is as close to the perfect disease as you can get...**

• It settles at the weakest point in each particular body
• Therefore, it can have different symptoms for most everyone that has it
• It causes the symptoms of - or causes - over 300 different diseases
• It is seldom diagnosed correctly therefore treatments are usually ineffective
• Most people can maintain for years and spend thousands for these ineffective treatments
• It is very contagious and can be passed on to their children, close friends & pets

- The name of the disease doesn't sound the least bit scary
- The standard myth is that you can only get it from one variety of the deer tick

From our personal experience and studies, Lyme Disease is very contagious and is not limited to certain rural areas of the country. It appears that a large portion of the population is already infected to some extent, and it can only gain momentum.

By now many people are infected who have never been in the woods / never been bitten and of course they have no clue to what is actually wrong.

All who have a sickness of any kind should check the symptom list to see if Lyme disease is a possibility.

**Lyme Disease is everywhere, but doctors are not paying attention to it.**

Many people are misdiagnosed as having something altogether different such as Crohn's disease, Fibromyalgia, or Lupus to name a few, but have the Lyme Disease bacteria as the basis of their sickness.

**List of some of the common misdiagnosed illnesses that seem to be caused by the Lyme disease spirochete:**

- Chronic Fatigue Syndrome
- Colitis
- Early ALS
- Early Alzheimer's disease
- Encephalitis
- Fibromyalgia
- Fifth's disease
- Gastro esophageal Reflux disease
- Infectious Cystitis
- Irritable Bowel Syndrome
- Juvenile Arthritis
- Joint Diseases/Joint Replacements
- Lupus
- Ménière's Syndrome
- Multiple Sclerosis
- Neuro-cognitive difficulties
- New-onset fatigue
- Osteoarthritis
- Prostatitis
- Psoriatic Arthritis
- Psychiatric disorders (bipolar, depression, etc.)
- Reynaud's Syndrome
- Reactive Arthritis

- Rheumatoid Arthritis
- Scleroderma
- Sjogren's Syndrome
- Sleep disorders
- Thyroid disease
- Widespread pain for no particular reason
- Various other illnesses with confusing symptoms

Source: http://canlyme.com/just-diagnosed/testing/common-misdiagnoses/

Following are the latest statistics I could find about the Lyme disease epidemic.

## Lyme disease Statistics

Lyme disease cases have been reported to have more than doubled in the US since the US Centers for Disease Control (CDC) began recording cases in 1999. In 2007, there were 28,222 cases of Lyme disease reported to the Center for Disease Control and Prevention (CDC) in the United States. (Just think of how many cases of Lyme were miss diagnosed and not reported!)

## Following are the latest statistics I could find about the Lyme disease epidemic

...9 cases per 100,000k populations

...2,287 cases per month

...77 per day

...3 people per hour

These statistics came from a recent newsletter on Lyme Disease from *www.genesis2church.org by Jim Humble*

This isn't even the tip of the iceberg...

The CDC has gone on record saying that they believe only 10-13% of Lyme disease cases are being reported to them.

So... multiply each statistic above by 10 or 12, and see how massive this epidemic truly is.

*(as reported in [http://mmsnews.is/newsletter/225-restoring-health-from-lyme-disease-is-completely-possible-05-01-2014](http://mmsnews.is/newsletter/225-restoring-health-from-lyme-disease-is-completely-possible-05-01-2014))*

**Many experts believe 300,000 people per year in the US are being infected with this disease.**

If we follow the CDC's own under-reported criteria, 270,222 cases is the reality for 2007

Now, think about all of the other diseases an insect can transmit along with Lyme disease... The insect can be a mosquito, as in yellow fever or dengue fever; a flea, as in bubonic plague; a tick or any other biting insect, as in Lyme disease; or a louse, as in trench fever.

Babesiosis as caused by microscopic parasites that infect red blood cells and are spread by certain ticks, Ehrlichiosis - flu-like the symptoms, Rocky Mountain spotted fever, Bartonella - cat scratch disease ... The magnitude and variety of this epidemic is unknown. These infections are known as co-infections to Lyme.

Reported Cases of Lyme in the United States:

Lyme Disease Statistics are still under-reported.

You will notice from this chart that Lyme disease far surpasses the totals of all the other diseases they try to scare us with and there's not a peep from the news media's talking heads about this epidemic. (Lyme is being under reported.)

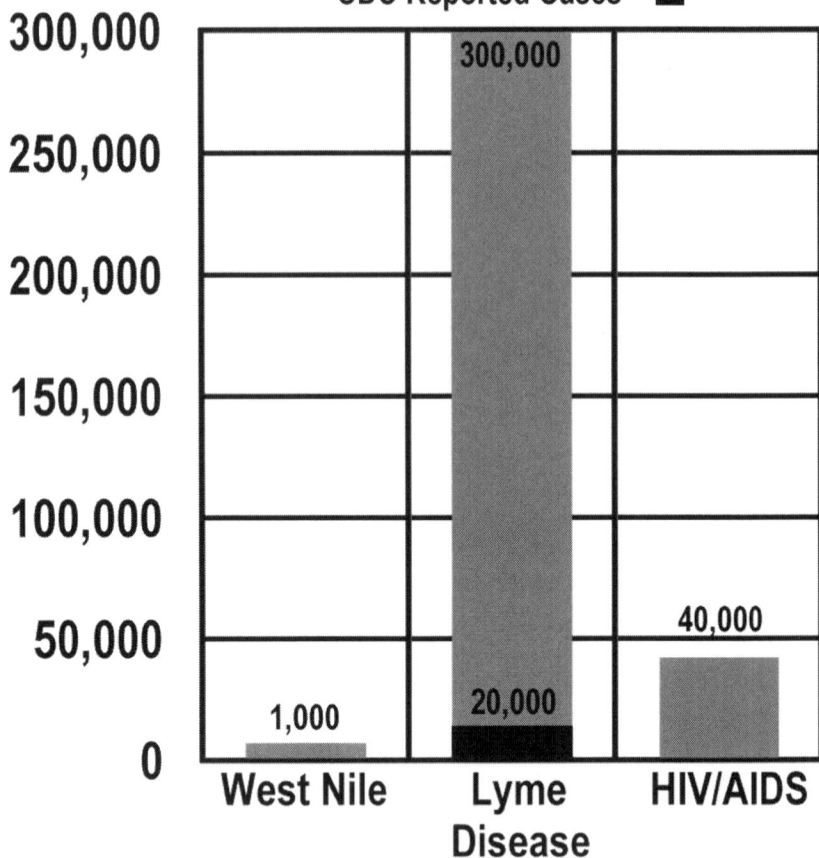

United States of America
CDC Reported Cases = ■

| | 300,000 |
| | 250,000 |
| | 200,000 |
| | 150,000 |
| | 100,000 |
| 40,000 | 50,000 |
| 1,000 | 20,000 | 0 |
| West Nile | Lyme Disease | HIV/AIDS |

# Chapter 3:

## *The Lyme Equation*

# Synopsis

You will learn why Lyme is called a vector-borne disease as well as what some of the symptoms can be and the reaction the doctors may have when you explain your symptoms to them.

How stress factors into the symptoms of Lyme disease and why one of the most inexpensive treatments will give you the best chance so far of success.

# The Lyme Equation

Spirochete Borrelia burgdorferi sensu lato complex is the official name of the spiral shaped bacteria causing Lyme disease. Lyme is the principal and most numerous disease of the total vector-borne illnesses found in the Northern hemisphere of the world.

## What is "Vector-borne disease"?

It is an illness caused by an infectious microbe that can be transmitted to people by biting insects. Arthropods (insects) or arachnids (spiders or others with 8 legs) are those which most commonly serve as vectors as listed below:

1.) blood sucking insects such as, fleas, lice, biting flies mosquitoes and bugs, and

2.) arachnids such as ticks, mites and spiders.

The term "vector" refers to any arthropod that transmits a disease through insect feeding activity. Lyme is not only a vector-borne disease but can be passed person to person, to children, pets and others by contact.

Lyme disease is by far the most prominent and it counts for more than 95% of the vector borne cases of illness in the country. Lyme disease has far surpassed AIDS as one of the fastest growing infectious epidemics in the United States, with an expense to society of over $1 billion annually.

## Lyme Disease Symptoms

Lyme disease will affect multiple body systems and cause a wide range of symptoms. But not all people will suffer all symptoms. The incubation period from infection is around two weeks usually but can be shorter or even longer. It can hide in the body for years without noticeable symptoms and after a stressful situation, cause so many conflicting symptoms at once that the doctor believes you are a nut case and recommends a couch doctor (psychologist, psychiatrist, ect...).

## The early infection location or contact area

The early localized infection is where Lyme disease didn't yet spread throughout your body. The only area is where the infection has first contacted the skin. The classic sign of early infection symptom is a circular red colour around the bite (if from the insect), the rash is red, could be target like and may be warm, itch some, but is in fact generally painless.

People can also suffer fever, malaise, and other flu like symptoms, headache, muscle soreness, tender, aching, throbbing, burning, and gnawing pain. Also, Lyme disease can progress to later stages in patients who haven't developed a rash, a target-shaped sore or "bulls-eye" patch or any redness around the bite.

**Early disseminated infections:**

Within two days to three weeks after the onset of local infections the bacteria may begin to spread out throughout your blood stream, tissue and bones. Stress might cause almost dormant bacteria to circulate to other places in the body. The symptoms are weakness, pain in the joints, muscles, tendons, also dizziness, vertigo and sometimes heart palpitations. Signs of early disseminated infections can also be a purplish lump that develops on the ear lobe, nipple or scrotum.

**Late disseminated infections:**

After a few months the untreated patient can develop severe and chronic symptoms that affect many parts of the body; this also includes the brain, the nerves, the eyes, joints and even the heart. Many of these symptoms may become permanent if left untreated.

Victims of Lyme will find their access to simple, often used, memories is intermittent. The way this sometimes shows up for me is: "I suddenly can't spell some simple word I've written thousands of times until I find a spelling book and re-boot my brain."

## Your body has an electrical charge

As I understand it from my studies all the necessary minerals and bacteria, which probiotics replenish and come from naturally grown foods, carry the same electrical charge as the body.

On the other hand, all the other stuff (critters such as bad bacteria, viruses, and their waste material, and toxic heavy metals) carry an opposite electrical charge.

What if you took an alterative health remedy that was electrically attracted to invasive bacteria, and their waste material? After a few days or weeks, what if you felt better?

**Chlorine Dioxide** carries the same electrical charge as the body, so it instantly goes after and neutralizes anything opposingly charged, such as heavy metals, critters or the critter's waste materials that it comes in contact with. The Chlorine Dioxide is destroyed along with the toxins it neutralizes. Chlorine Dioxide only remains active in the body for about one hour, so it's most effective if used every hour.

Your body's immune system already makes some of the Chlorine Dioxide so in effect you are simply strengthening the immune system's response to invaders.

One young man 22 years old took the solution for his allergies and experienced a huge boost in energy. He took a bottle home to Hawaii and gave the water purifier drops to his bed-ridden grandmother. After a few days on the solution, she could turn over in the bed by herself.

We personally used Chlorine Dioxide to get rid of Lyme disease we'd had almost ten years.

To kill Lyme, it makes sense to me for others to also use Chlorine Dioxide (water purifier also called MMS) because it works instantly, electrically, and even mechanically. The Chlorine dioxide reacts when it comes into contact with oppositely charged bacteria. It destroys them in moments. They don't have time to run and hide, or morph into another form to camouflage their presence. WP seems to electrically destroy them and instantly do the job.

## The American Diet Was Killing Us

In addition to using the MMS / WP to kill the colonies of spirochetes invading our bodies, we changed our diet to eating mostly organic foods, raw and slightly cooked. We seldom eat anything from the middle of a grocery store anymore. That means we do not go near the canned, boxed, or already prepared groceries. By eliminating artificial flavors, MSG, artificial sugars, high fructose corn syrup, Nitrates, preservatives to keep out mold, food colorings, and other chemical additives from your diet, you're helping cleanse your body to live a healthier and more natural lifestyle. Have you heard that your body is a self-healing machine? Your natural immunity increases when you remove additives. Start reading labels.

We also quit eating breads and pasta except maybe once a month. We did not go to extremes, and we did study the non-inflammation diet and the anti-Candida way of eating.

Hardly any sugar except raw sugar and no artificial sugars at all will be found in our house. We made small changes by adding even more micronutrient content (eating food with life force energy) and made major changes in the kind of food we brought home.

We grow a large organic garden with tomatoes, onions, carrots, beets, potatoes, cucumbers, peas, green beans, artichokes and many different kinds of squash. If gardening is not feasible for your lifestyle, go to the local farmers markets to stock up.

Fresh grass fed beef is also available locally if you search. There are three essential amino acids found in beef that are not readily available any other way. We added some grass fed beefsteaks to our diet. All these food changes help the immune system recover your health and stamina.

The most important building block to recovery is adding real live nutrition and developing a mindset to love your body enough to insist on feeding it food that is not dead, over processed, and full of additives with names you cannot even pronounce.

**Love your body into wellness! Love heals!**

When we come to the point of view that *everything is a blessing*, we are no longer fighting a disease. In the book "Power Verses Force" it ranks a person's spiritual progress at 500 when *everything is a blessing.*

Keeping your energy up and being optimistic about the outcome is important. There are many cases where a placebo has instantly healed a person. How can this happen?

The feeling of --"why me?" will attract more feelings of being a victim. We are not taught about the Law of Attraction in government school. All of the more successful people have read "Think and Grow Rich" by Napoleon Hill. If a person wants to be successful in any endeavor they must control the mind and get it on board by thinking only thoughts that are beneficial.

NOTES:

# Chapter 4:

## *Impossible or Incurable?*

# Synopsis

Learn how we found the simple way to kick most of the "incurable diseases," how this interesting product was discovered, the three things it does, and...

Public proof it does things considered impossible by conventional medicine.

There is also a list of different names used for this product that neutralizes the spirochetes. This will clear up any confusion.

# Impossible or Incurable?

We got real lucky!
After trying several recommended products that were supposed to control Lyme disease and only slowing it down a little, a friend told us about a water purifying product. We used it to kick Lyme bacteria out of our bodies, and not just to control it.

Many Lyme patients have been told that it is incurable. Well, with conventional medications and drugs that might be so.

**The secret we used to kill the Lyme disease spirochetes is Chlorine Dioxide.**

In this application, it is most commonly called MMS (Master Mineral Solution) on the Internet. It costs around $25.00 USD for a year's supply of these drops. Only three drops are used for each treatment. A person must work up to taking three drops an hour for 8 hours a day. It's very efficient, but it's doubtful this solution will ever become mainstream because there's not enough profit in it for the pharmaceutical companies.

This water purification solution has been on the market for about 80 years as a water purifier. It gets rid of, rather than just managing a disease. It kills the bacteria, virus and fungus.

## What is this master mineral solution?

Basically, MMS is a water purifier, and the chemical name is Chlorine Dioxide.

To kill Lyme it makes sense to me to use Chlorine Dioxide (Water purifier also called MMS) because it is electrically drawn to oppositely charged items in the body and when they contact, they both go out of existence and become inert waste material and are naturally eliminated.

Jim Humble found, out of necessity, that Chlorine Dioxide tablets (water purification) not only killed bacteria in your drinking water while he was in the Venezuelan jungle, but worked to kill Malaria bugs inside a human body' blood stream as well.

They were way back in the jungle at least five days by runner from conventional malaria medicine when his survey team got Malaria. He was the only one that hadn't got sick, so he figured the water purifier he was drinking might help them. As it turned out, it did help them get over the sickness almost immediately. This process became his ministry and since he is an engineer he beefed it up to work better than the hiking and camping tablets most people take. He invented a two-bottle set of solutions for you to do it yourself.

**How is chlorine dioxide generated?**

You make Chlorine Dioxide at home on your kitchen counter top. You just combine two items:

1.  In a dry glass put one or more drops of Sodium Chlorite 28% (usually comes in a 4 oz green bottle with a dropper top).
2.  Add a matching number of drops of 50% Citric Acid* and swirl together, wait 20-30 seconds to activate.  The mixture will change from a clear to yellow color. Fill the glass with water. Use immediately or cap tightly.  The sooner you use it, the better it works.
3.  For activator you can use a food acid. It requires five drops of fresh lemon juice for each 1 drop of Sodium Chlorite.  This method takes

three minutes to activate because the acid is weaker.

4. Do not use metal containers.

How to make the activator if you did not purchase a set of bottles.

>*The 50% citric acid liquid is made by filling any size container ½ full of Citric acid powder and filling it up with distilled water. (Keep this Simple formula and you have a 50/50% protocol to make the activator.) The 50/50 activates MMS in 20-30 seconds to make the Chlorine Dioxide.

**I believe this CD solution was discovered in Russia in the 1800's.** It has been used to purify community water supplies for over 80 years, especially in Europe, and has been sold as a handy kit for campers and explorers. It's been known to kill most all pathogens so it doesn't matter what disease you have been diagnosed with. It'll probably eliminate most bacteria, fungus, mold, and viruses in a person's body for less than 50 cents a week.

Homeland Security has used it to kill Anthrax. It has also been used to kill black fungus in the homes flooded in hurricanes. It is pumped into homes as a CD gas and left over night. It is used in meat packing plants to wash down carcasses to kill bacteria. It does not have to be washed off.

**The Chlorine Dioxide (CD)** in solution is a light to dark yellow colored liquid oxidizing agent and it has a-chlorine-like smell. It is also a gas and the fumes are yellowish green color. It has nothing in common with the Chlorine cities put into drinking water to kill bacteria. Well, both of them are bleach, but that's all they have in common. CD is healthy for us.

**Different names for this water purifier can be confusing.**

1. Jim Humble's Master Mineral Supplement
2. Sodium Chlorite 28%
3. MMS
4. Miracle Mineral Solution
5. Chlorine Dioxide (CD)
6. Water Purification Drops
7. Water Purification Solution
8. Chlorine Dioxide pills

If you choose to take the water purifier start real slow, real slow. There is no rush! In fact, the worse your sickness the less you use to start so you don't kill so much stuff that the body gets sick trying to get rid of the trash (called a Herxheimer reaction). I've seen people who will activate only one drop and put it in a 16 oz plastic drinking bottle of distilled water. They might drink little sips all day long just acclimatizing their body to it.

**This Water purifier only does three things:**

**1) Kills pathogens**
**2) Oxides their poop**
**3) Oxides heavy metals**

The Water purifier does not heal the body. It does not cure disease. It helps the immune system kill pathogens and helps clean up the body. Only you can heal your body.

After 60+ years of use in the U.S. food industry and numerous research projects proving the safety of Chlorine Dioxide. Even as the Homeland Security has used CD against killer-bacteria in so-called terrorist attacks, etc. The FDA has now decided it's unsafe for us to use it. Instead of people using a proven safe product that costs $25.00 for up to a year's supply, they encourage us to use drugs developed by their Pharmaceutical Corporation buddies that cost several thousand dollars for about a year's supply and most all drugs have harsh side effects. Chlorine Dioxide used as described by Jim Humble has no side effects.

Even if the FDA so-called approved drugs really did as good a job as this simple immune booster (MMS), couldn't the extra thousands be better spent by us -- as the down payment on a house, new cars, etc. We could all use the extra money to live better and have more fun.

Isn't it odd that a supposedly independent government agency such as the F.D.A. does everything to support the food and drug industries that they are supposed to protect us from?

When 10 yrs ago Jim Humble discovered that Chlorine Dioxide would kill all the Malaria in a person's blood in less than 24 hours, then why is Malaria still considered "incurable" and can only be "managed" by the health authorities?

**Early in 2013 a local Red Cross branch in Uganda did a full-fledged scientific test on 154 random people who were first tested and proved to have Malaria.**

Within 48 hours all 154 of the Malaria patients were tested to be absolutely clear of Malaria. Understand this usually life-long disease was not just "managed" but clear gone; publicly proving Jim Humble's claims about Chlorine Dioxide are 100% correct. (Google Youtube.com video https://www.youtube.com for proof: *Red Cross Cures 154 Malaria Cases in Uganda.*)

Do you think the benevolent International Red Cross will admit it? Would their corporate drug buddies stop donating to the Red Cross if they did admit it?

Malaria causes more than three hundred million acute illnesses and kills at least one million people every year.

It is estimated that 10 million people around the world have used this water purifier despite the smear campaign, and misinformation corporate paid bloggers have posted on the Internet about it being only a bleach and dangerous.

Dangerous? We're talking about using drops, not large amounts! No, it is not dangerous; my wife and I took it everyday for near two years, getting over this disease.

Despite the anti MMS blogging,  there are hundreds of thousands of positive testimonials from people that have gotten rid of almost every kind of "incurable" disease including Malaria with Chlorine Dioxide.

(Note: If you spill or wipe some on your clothes it will change the color of the fabric.)

# Chapter 5:

## *Spirochetes and Drug Salesmen*

# Synopsis

In this chapter you will learn how the Spirochete type of bacteria may be the major cause of the huge rash of joint replacements we hear about most every day from people we know.

A little about why we have the "side effect" riddled care industry we have today.

Learn how the MDs became drug sales people.

# Spirochetes and Drug Salesmen

There's another aspect of spirochetes in general that's not usually addressed. They seem to congregate in joints and eat the cushioning out faster than the body can replace it. The usual diagnosis is – the joint is worn-out and must be replaced with a mechanical one that can't repair itself.

To me it makes more sense to evict the hungry little critters, eat a little healthier diet yourself, let the body do as it's designed to and build those joints back up.

Eat more live, fresh food – keep away from processed foods. Get on an anti-inflammatory diet. Just make 2 or 3 major changes at a time so as to not shock the body.

I recently talked to an acquaintance that had to have his artificial joint relined after 8 years. He wishes he hadn't let them do the surgery in the first place.

We have to remember those medical people are salesmen selling a $60,000+ job for which they get a commission. Very few salesmen would suggest a $25.00 natural remedy life-long fix alternative. You may not be aware of the history of so called main stream medicine. A very wealthy American family had huge interests in chemical corporations.

There was way more production capability than they were using. The family decided they needed more effective drug salesmen so they made large grants to medical schools to shape the education of those students. This way they were training them as drug salesmen.

Little by little the Rockefellers financially took over the medical schools, slowly changing the direction of healing away from natural remedies, and aiming the curriculums toward their advantage in pushing their pills by way of their huge grants. These graduating medical doctors really became drug salesmen.

The scheme worked so well that real healers are now called alternative. It does not hurt their campaign that the corporations have bought up almost all of the news media, TV stations, magazines and radio stations. They effectively control what articles get released as the "news" and we get only their side of their story.

That's a short version of how most of the world went from <u>healing</u> to <u>controlling</u> diseases and selling their corporate drugs.

**Sound like a fairy tale?**

You must understand the doctors are – for the most part – doing absolutely the best they can. They've been taken in by the scheme just like most of the rest of us. Many of them move into natural medicine or quit when the whole realization finally sinks in.

**Do we hear about this on the mighty news?**

Hardly! The news has all been bought up by the same interlocking corporations that own big pharmacies.

Don't believe this story? Look it up on the Internet; it is all available. Read "The Drug Story", and "The House of Rockefeller."

# Chapter 6:

## *What Can You Do?*

---

# Synopsis

In this chapter you will find out about some of the co-infections that may accompany the Lyme bacteria and about documented testing of many being treated for other diseases and actually have Lyme disease.

You will find a symptoms list to check yourself to see if Lyme is likely your problem.

More about ex-aerospace engineer Jim Humble who accidentally discovered how useful Chlorine Dioxide is for killing bacteria.

# What Can You Do?

One good reason to use a broad spectrum product like MMS (Water Purification Drops) to kick Lyme disease is because Lyme doesn't always get deposited into your body alone. Any biting insect can carry Lyme along with several other little-known buddies.

**Three of the most common co-infections are:**

- Babesia,

- Bartonella and

- Mycoplasma Fermentans

Any of these along with Lyme will confuse the diagnosis even more, along with making it even more unlikely that a focused antibiotic will clear your infections.

Even though it's seldom acknowledged, Lyme disease and its buddies are the most common diseases in the northern hemisphere.

The myth the medical mainstream continues to mouth is that it's only a tick-borne disease. Doctors generally ask if you've been camping, hiking, hunting in the woods, etc. If you haven't, then you couldn't possibly have Lyme disease.

As far back as 1995 transmission of the disease has been clearly documented after bites by mites, fleas, mosquitoes, spiders and ticks.

> Syphilis or The Great Imitator is caused by a bacteria called Treponeum palladium. T. palladium belongs to a group of bacteria that are cork-screw serpentine shaped and are referred to as spirochetes. Bacteria in this group cause Lyme disease, Relapsing Fever and Leptospirosis. They all have a three-phase life cycle like Syphilis. from website - *http://filmtecmembrane.blogspot.com/2011/0 8/syphilis-bacterial-infection-called.html*

**Dr. Lida Mattman**, Author of "Cell Wall Deficient Forms: Stealth Pathogens (CRC Press 2000)", has been able to recover live Lyme Spirochetes from mosquitoes, fleas, mites, semen, urine, blood, Tears and Spinal fluid. In 1995, Dr. Mattman obtained positive cultures of Lyme (Borreliosis) from 43 of 47 chronically ill persons.

• All 8 of the cases of Parkinson's disease she tested actually had Lymes.

- 21 cases of Amyotrophic Lateral Sclerosis (Als) and every tested case of Alzheimer's all were actually Lyme disease.

- She later obtained cultures from 25 patients with fibromyalgia; all were positive for the cell wall deficient form of the Lyme Spirochete.

- Since most antibiotics kill bacteria by breaking down the cell wall, they have very little effect on your critters without a cell wall to break down. Dr. Lida Mattman was a biology Professor and a bacteriologist. In the jelly wall stage of the bacteria antiboitics will not work!

Lyme disease is just like its sister disease Syphilis in the fact that it is highly contagious.

Since the bacteria can be found in all the body fluids including saliva and tears. It could be transferred by a kiss, drinking and eating from the same utensils. It could come out of a skin lesion or scrape. A dog licking you or your kids can transport the bacteria. It can be airborne, too, from a sneeze, cough, etc...

It's very easy for a whole family to be infected, even though, each may show entirely different symptoms.

If you look at it under a powerful enough microscope, you will see the corkscrew bacteria that looks like tiny snakes. The evil culprit of Lyme disease, Borrelia Burgdorferi looks like a coiled snake, as well as in syphilis.

Syphilis is acquired through contact with infected mucus membranes, body fluids, etc. Parts that can be infected on our body are the mouth and lips, vagina, penis and rectum. The eye can also be infected and for many years when syphilis was a bigger problem all newborns were treated with silver nitrate in each eye to prevent infection. Therefore, Syphilis and Lyme disease can be acquired through unprotected oral, vaginal and rectal sex and during birth if the mother has an active infection. Somehow it is very difficult to identify those microorganisms that look like little snakes.

Lyme disease is nearly impossible to be diagnosed accurately because the two best tests for the disease are no longer available (i.e., Dr. Lida Mattman's Blood Culture Technique and Dr. JoAnne Whitaker's Q-RIBb test). The Lyme bacteria are most easily grown in a laboratory in an isolation chamber where the oxygen level is very low. These tests were foolproof because growing spirochaetes out of the blood or visualising pieces of spirochaetes in blood samples constitutes undeniable proof of diagnosis.

## Why did these tests never become mainstream?

That is a good question and deserves to be answered by the AMA and the FDA. These two tests were very accurate, and the results were easily cultured in a laboratory. Why are these tests, not in full use?

Remember any body fluid, even a sneeze, from an infected person or animal, can transmit Lyme disease!

Millions of people are infected and most don't even have a clue that's what's wrong!

What if your dog has a deer tick bite and licks your baby in the mouth? Lyme disease could be transmitted that easy.

**The good news is the Water purifier, made from Sodium Chlorite and Citric acid usually kicks it in a few months.**

Why not just try it?

When you begin to feel better, you will know you are on the right track.

## What are the symptoms of Lyme Disease?

I had several of those symptoms that indicated that it was probable that I had Lyme disease even before I was tested.

Check the list below to find out how many of the following symptoms you have. These are **common symptoms of people who have Lyme disease to some degree.**

## Circle the numbers that apply.

1   Unusual chills, fevers, sweats or flushing
2   Unusual weight loss or gain
3.  Unusual hair loss
4.  Tiredness, lack of stamina, fatigue
5.  Swollen Glands
6.  Throat sore
7.  Pelvic Pain or testicle pain
8.  Bladders irritable or poor function
9.  Unusual menstrual irregularity
10. Sexual – loss of libido, dysfunction
11. Abdominal pains or poor digestion
12. Regularity changes – diarrhea, constipation
13. Sore ribs or pain in chest

14. Pulse skips
15. Pain or swelling in joints: Which ones?
16. Breast pain, unexplained milk production
17. Joint & back stiffness
18. Muscles twitching: especially in face
19. Hear/feel cracking when turning neck
20. Cramps or pain in muscles
21. Neck pain or stiffness
22. Headache
23. Blurry vision, sensitive to light
24. Ear pain, sensitive to sounds
25. Occasional Vertigo, poor balance
26. Sudden need to lie down or sit
27. Suddenly unable to spell simple words
28. Short term memory poor
29. Concentration difficult
30. Getting lost, hard to find car in parking lot
31. Mood swings, anger, depression
32. Sleep disturbances – Wake early etc.
33. Tremors
34. Swollen tissue, rashes, oozing fluid
35. More sensitive to alcoholic drinks, exagerated, worst hangover
36. Knee, hip, shoulder joint replacement
37. Sleep Apnea
38. Muscles twisting and pulling in late stages

Several of these numbers circled might indicate, you should take serious steps to get your health back on track.

**Getting back to kicking Lyme disease:**
> My hands were hurting and had been swollen for two years so I couldn't close them. After three weeks, use of the water purifier (Chlorine Dioxide) the swelling was gone in my hands, and I could use them to grasp things again. My overall health continued to get better at a kind of progressive rate for the next several months and was completely over the various symptoms in a year.

I continued regular use of Chlorine Dioxide for about another year to make sure. I went on the maintenance of 6 to 10 drops a day.

Since then, I've talked to dozens of people who've spent thousands of dollars and 20 to 30 years trying to get rid of Lyme disease with few results if any from using traditional treatments.

It's well known that our bodies are 70% to 80% water, so it makes perfect sense to purify that water. I understand our body's immune system makes a small amount of this Chlorine Dioxide - the purifier already. We're simply helping our immune system do a better job in spite of todays greatly expanded pollution. I consider it a natural way to improve my body's resistance to pathogens and clean house Water Purifier is easy to make -- just combine two products: Sodium Chlorite and Citric Acid are combined in a small 1 to 1 drop solution at the time of use to form Chlorine Dioxide. Most people will work up to 3 drops an hour for 8 hours a day. At times we were taking 30 drops a day.

**There are only three changes water purifier can make:**
1. Kill Pathogens
2. Oxidize the pathogen's waste material (they are not house broke, you know!)
3. Oxidize heavy metals.

During this oxidation process, the Water Purifier is also destroyed, and it most all happens within the 1st hour of use. For this reason, it's recommended that some WP be taken every hour to keep a pressure on whatever you're trying to kick.

I combined the drops in the dry glass for 20-30 seconds. Next I simply pour ½ glass of water into the activated drops to dilute. The drops are clear when they are put in the dry glass and change to a yellow color after the 20 to 30 seconds of activation.

Note: The drops must be combined in a dry container, and you wait 20-30 seconds before the water is added. You should be activating only a few drops at a time, not the whole bottle.

Since they are so efficient at killing pathogens - the worse the problem, the fewer the drops, you start with, so you won't kill too much trash at once and overload the bodies elimination systems. You might start with only one drop from each bottle and see how that goes. Put the combined drops in a 16 oz drinking bottle and fill with distilled water. Keep the lid on tightly so the CD gas will not excape I would just drink a little of that each hour all the first day. The MMS Protocol 1000 calls for working up to 3 drops each hour and repeat every hour for 8 hours a day.

I'm a researcher and a student of life experiences. I'm not a doctor and not even a Veterinarian so I can't make any recommendation for you to use the product or not.

It worked for us!

The book that explains it all is "The Master Mineral Solution of the Third Millennium" by ex Aero-Space engineer Jim Humble.

**Jim accidentally discovered it would cure Malaria while working in the South American jungle.**

Being an avid researcher he spent several years experimenting with Chlorine Dioxide after his return so he could understand what was happening. He immediately knew if he tried to patent and make money from his discoveries the Big Pharmacy would swat him like a bug. Instead he slowly slipped it into common use all over the world at his own expense and with the help of friends so the people wouldn't be deprived of yet another simple inexpensive healing agent.

Jim still spends thousands of dollars travelling all over the world introducing MMS discreetly to small groups of sick people. Malaria alone kills at least a million people every year in the tropics, many of them children.

**Remember, One branch of the Red Cross did a 154-person test in Uganda and proved Jim Humble's claim that all were cured.**

In the blood it's easier to kick out the critters than getting rid of those that scatter throughout the body tissue, connective tissue, cartilage and bones. Malaria is a disease of the blood that is caused by the Plasmodium parasite, which is transmitted from person to person by a particular type of mosquito.

This is why curing Malaria - a blood disease - is quicker than treating Lyme disease where the spirochetes are in the deep tissue, joints and bore into the bones. The water purifier solution easily and quickly goes into the blood system right after it leaves the stomach. Healing Malaria (killing the Plasmodium parasite) with the water purifier may only take 24 hours to a couple days.

**Lyme Disease Tests Cost Hundreds of Dollars**

You can get expensive tests at several hundred dollars so you can brag about the brand name of your sickness or spend $25.00 for a set of WP bottles and personally take responsibility for testing yourself and taking care of your problem. Do the $25 Lyme test!

If the problems start to go away after trying the WP drops for just 3 weeks, who cares what the official brand name of the disease was? I consider the $500 I spent on tests a total waste of money.

The symptoms list would have done that at zero cost - just go down the list; check off the symptoms you are experiencing.

We used the MMS (water purifier - WP) to kill the Lyme spirochete and are forever grateful to Jim Humble for being one of the few inventors who really understands how the Earth's greedy health care system works. He knew a simple inexpensive remedy would never be tolerated by big business and their captive F.D.A. So Humble followed his heart and gave it directly to the people.

Learn more about the Lyme Treatment -
http://bit.ly/Lymetreatment

Herb "Roi" Richards is an internationally published writer who is well versed in Alternative Health and well-being.

For more information visit:
http://www.fibromyalgialupuslyme.com/

NOTES:

23388072R00037

Printed in Great Britain
by Amazon